Introduction

Welcome and congratulations on taking the first step to having the body you want. As a Trainer I have spent many years trying and testing numerous fat loss strategies with my clients and, of course, myself. I believe the weight loss program that you are about to undertake is the simplest, fastest and healthiest plan to lose those unwanted kilos. The following approach will get you in shape and on time, but it does require discipline, determination, and unwavering commitment.

Most diets have a failure rate of 90-95%. This is not because they are ineffective but because the dieting strategy is unsustainable, too restrictive and quite simply not-fun. There's a smarter way to achieve your weight loss goals. In the time it takes for you to finish reading this book, you will have all the tools and knowledge you need not only to lose weight and look phenomenal for your event, but also to maintain your goal weight for life.

Deadline Dieting lays out a dieting strategy which will easily become part of your lifestyle. Why? Because our natural eating patterns are truly one of periods of feasting and fasting. Times of plenty were scarce in our past and obesity has never been so prevalent as it is now. So, now that you've made the decision to change your body and your life, what do you need? Well that's the beauty of the "Deadline Dieting" plan. You don't need any special equipment. You don't even need a gym membership. There are no special health supplements or pills to take. All you need is an open mind and a willingness to restructure your eating times.

Now I'm sure you're already aware of all the benefits of a lean and healthy body, but, just in case, this is a taste of what awaits you on the other side:

You're going to break necks. New body, new you, new attitude. All that combined is going to stop people in their tracks. People will treat you differently. Yes it's true, attractive people do receive favourable treatment (fair or not, it happens)

You will notice you have more energy. Weight loss has profound beneficial effects on all aspects of health and increased energy is a major bonus!

You're simply going to feel great. You will receive that precious form of confidence that only comes from achievement. You will also likely experience better mental acuity and notice positive benefits to many seemingly unrelated areas of life.

Losing weight is more of a mental challenge than it is a physical challenge. This will be a repeating theme throughout this book as having the right mindset is truly the difference between success and failure. No matter what weight loss plan you undertake there are going to be moments of extreme discomfort and hunger. But remember, that discomfort is only temporary and it too shall pass. The weight loss and health benefits will stay, making it more than worth it.

It's a cliche but it's true "Self-improvement begins at the end of your comfort zone." I therefore encourage you to embrace any discomfort you experience throughout this plan. Look upon discomfort more as a signal that life-changing results are just around the corner. Befriend discomfort and it will do you a world of good.

There are three very important tips I want to give you before we start this journey together.

Deadline Dieting Tip #1: Beware of Critical & Negative People

People who are not supportive of your weight loss goals and techniques have the potential to derail your success before you even get started.

Our mind is a delicate thing and must be fed positive thoughts just like our bodies should be fuelled by healthy foods to accomplish our goals. Allowing people the opportunity to voice their negative opinions often plants seeds of doubt in our minds. During the tougher periods of weight loss, our minds will play tricks on us and search for excuses to breakdown and give in to temptation. This is when any doubts you are harbouring can gain strength and surface, potentially derailing any success you've had or were going to have.

When it comes to diet and nutrition, everyone has an opinion on the right and wrong way of doing things. If given the opportunity, your closest friends and co-workers will turn into weight-loss gurus.

These people can unknowingly be very damaging to your goals. They can also directly affect your weight loss through the extra stress they cause you, mentally and emotionally. Our bodies have evolved to handle stress in a very specific way, and the increased release of stress hormones can cause your weight loss to slow down or stop.

Talking publicly about nutrition and weight loss strategies can be as controversial as discussing religion and, therefore, is a subject best left untouched. I tell all my clients not to engage in conversations regarding weight loss or nutrition to avoid negative feedback and conversations that could steer them from their course.

I know that once the weight starts dropping off and the results become more visible it will be very tempting to want to share your newfound knowledge and experience. It's human nature to be proud of your victories and to want to help your loved ones do the same.

However, I caution you to think twice before you speak. One small battle doesn't mean the war has been won so you don't want to get ahead of yourself. You also do not want to invite the critics to comment and hinder any progress you've made. Finally, most people do not learn deeply nor develop deep appreciation for things freely given. That learning and appreciation is only gained by investing of themselves, their time, their effort, and their money. If they don't earn it, they won't learn it. If you try to give someone the verbal cliff notes of this plan, it may not translate and there will be vital pieces to the puzzle missing. Therefore, I encourage you to share your copy of this book with them.

A picture is worth a thousand words so let your visual results speak for themselves. Surround yourself with positive and supportive people that will help push your progress forward and I promise you, your weight loss journey will be much easier and more enjoyable.

Deadline Dieting Tip #2: Leave everything you know about Diet, Fitness and Nutrition at the door.

There is an abundance of bad science, outdated nutrition rules, and misinformation readily available and permeating the diet and nutrition world. Every nutrition and weight loss rule you've ever heard is only true within a specific context. For example, to say that high fat intake is bad would depend on the context. Keeping fat intake low on a high-carb calorie-controlled diet may be a good idea, but it would be a bad idea on a very low-carb diet.

So start from a clean slate of knowledge, and follow only the guidelines laid out in this one eating plan. Do not mix and match different dietary approaches. In my experience, 99% of diets do work, but only if done within the guidelines specifically outlined by the plan. So commit to following this eating plan only and do it 100% - not 99% or 50%. Provided you have no underlying health issues, it will be impossible not to reach your goals.

Deadline Dieting Tip #3: Stay Hungry

Stay hungry for results, and stay motivated. Success is dependent on a dedicated single-mindedness. It's that feeling, that state of mind where all you can focus on is achieving that one goal and everything else is in the world becomes background noise! Allow yourself to experience this state and become a little self-involved in order to achieve this one goal. Set a goal weight and stick to it. Fully invest and immerse yourself in the process of achieving your goal. Keep your standards high, and discipline yourself to not allow any exceptions or give in to any of your usual excuses.

A common occurrence for many people on a weight loss plan is to start out super strong with 110% enthusiasm and effort. Then, after seeing some fantastic results (usually around the 4-6 week mark), they relax their efforts and return to old eating habits without ever truly achieving their goal. This, in turn, brings them right back to where they started and the vicious cycle of dieting begins again.

Fat loss is a marathon not a sprint. This means consistency over a longer period of time is what really matters to get you to your weight loss goals. While following my eating plan, pay close attention to your thoughts about eating and food. You're not alone in your struggles, and you owe it to yourself not to give in. Allowing yourself to think thoughts like "I'll just try a little bit" will not serve you, and only whets the appetite for more of that food. Thoughts repeated become habits and habits are hard to break.

Recognise and stop the following common thought patterns: These will derail your success and make your weight loss journey much more difficult.

"I've been good all week I deserve a treat!" (It's fine to treat yourself, but not with food. Treat yourself with non-food items until you reach your goal weight.)

"I'm nearly at my goal weight so I don't need to be as strict!" (This is when you should be at your strictest as this is where most people give up.)

"It's a waste not to finish it – there are people in the world starving!" (This is something our parents ingrained into our heads as children to scare us into finishing our vegetables.) This is faulty logic and, as adults, we should understand by now the reasons we need to eat healthily. World starvation is an issue, but best solved in ways other than eating everything on your plate if you're already satiated. Not finishing your plate is far better and healthier for you in the long run than eating past your fullness signals. Get in tune with your body. It will tell you when it's full.)

"Well I've blown my diet now so I may as well eat anything." (A minor slip up every now and then on your journey can be expected, but don't destroy all of the week's hard work by letting it get out of control.)

"Just this one time." (This gives power to the next "one time" to happen so don't start the cycle.)

"I'll start the diet tomorrow." ("Tomorrow" is just another excuse to eat what you want today. This thought pattern that will not serve you in the long run.)

"I've had a really bad day so I'm going to break my diet." (Food should never be used as an emotional band-aid.)

These are just a handful of the lies we tell to allow ourselves to deviate from our plans and goals. If we allow ourselves to give in to these thoughts once, then we will likely give in to these thoughts in the future. These thoughts will only make your journey more difficult and even longer than when you started.

Nothing worth achieving is easy so take this seriously and be extremely strict with yourself. Maintain a healthy and disciplined mindset, and make this the last weight loss plan you will ever use.
Now, let's get started!

Chapter 1: The Concept

The "Deadline Dieting" approach is a simple, extremely effective, and a safe way to drop kilos fast. First, let's cover some basics. I will try to keep the biology lessons to a minimum, but I encourage you to do your own research for a deeper understanding of the principles outlined here.

Ask a child how to lose weight, and they will quite simply tell you to "eat less". Ask an adult this same question, and you could get a thousand different answers, including:

Eat breakfast
Eat small meals every 2 – 3 hours
Eat low-fat meals
Eat a big breakfast, a medium lunch, and a small dinner
Count calories
Eat more whole grains and vegetables
Eat more fibre
Don't eat sugar
Cut out dairy
Cut carbohydrates
Eat low-glycaemic foods
Skip breakfast
Exercise more

The list goes on and on.

The world of nutrition and dieting is full of contradicting advice and rules.

So let's keep things simple – every single diet or weight loss plan that has ever worked has one thing in common. The person dieting eats less. It's not rocket science. It is scientific fact. You must eat less food than what your body needs to lose weight.

All those jiggly bits that we affectionately call love handles, rolls, extra padding, are really just stored energy (stored food). This is how I want you to think of losing weight. You have a choice, you can either use the food you put in your mouth for energy, or you can burn the food already stored on your body.

Fat tissue is extremely energy dense, and is a perfectly, healthy energy source. In fact, there are many instances of people surviving for great lengths of time on nothing but water, some vitamins and minerals while functioning quite normally in their everyday activities. One such case is an Irishman known only as Mr. A B.

In 1965, Mr. A B checked himself into the Department of Medicine at the Royal Infirmary in Dundee, advising the University hospital staff that he was sick of being overweight and that he was going to fast no matter what they said so they may as well monitor him. The hospital staff did monitor him, and, after 3 days of continuous fasting, checked Mr. A B out. Mr. A B continued his fast outside of the hospital, and, with weekly check-ins by hospital staff, he ended up fasting for a total of 382 continuous days. His weight dropped from 207 kg to 82 kg, and, even more surprising, he was able to maintain most of his weight loss after 5 years, only gaining 7 kg back. When questioned about his experience, Mr. A B spoke of the fast as effortless to endure with normal energy levels. As a result of the weight loss, all of Mr. A B's health markers significantly improved. Now, I am not recommending this extreme a fast, but it is important for you to understand that the human body will adapt and survive perfectly fine off its own body fat stores. The human body is a remarkable thing. It is our mind and our will that we need to retrain. An average 70 kg male has approximately 1,904 calories of energy stored as glycogen or stored carbohydrates and about 95,238 calories stored as body fat. That's a lot of food!

So, how do we access our fat stores and eat less without it being a major hassle?

Simple. We separate our day into a fasting period, where we don't consume any calories at all, and a feeding period. This is something we all naturally do anyway while we sleep. This is of course why breakfast is called "break-fast."

The Deadline Dieting plan pushes that fasting period to a minimum of 16 hours followed by an eating window of 8 hours. This sounds tougher than it actually is.

Your daily 16-hour fast can be quite easily achieved by skipping breakfast. For many, this style of eating will be quite effortless as they're not naturally hungry at breakfast.

Hang on....skip breakfast??!!! What nutritional heresy is this?! I will go into more detail later on why skipping breakfast is not only healthy but, also, a powerful fat-loss technique. There are many health benefits to fasting for 16 hours, but the one we're most interested in is the powerful fat loss effects.

Some may argue that, from an evolutionary point of view, this is how we've naturally evolved to eat. Historically, we would often go for periods of 24 hours or more without food so, anthropologically speaking, it makes sense.

Periods of fasting followed by periods of feasting were quite common. Up until recently, we have never lived in a time period where food was so readily available!

Our genetic makeup has not actually changed that much since our cave-dwelling days but our eating habits, the frequency of our meals, and the amount of food has changed and increased dramatically. It's not hard to see why those extra love handles have found a home around many a waist.

The "Deadline Dieting" plan has been formulated to use the foods and meal timings that we're best genetically suited to eat.

Chapter 2: It's the Hormones

Have you noticed that when you routinely eat meals at the same times, you will always be hungry at the exact same times? This phenomenon can be used to your advantage while losing weight. If you only eat once a day, then, once adapted, you will tend to only get hungry once a day. Bear in mind that we are discussing true physical hunger, not cravings or hunger from wanting or seeing food.

One of the major reasons we feel hungry at the same times each day is due to the hormone ghrelin, also known as "the hunger hormone". Ghrelin rises in anticipation of a meal and is in tune with your day-to-day meal pattern. So, yes, it is possible to train yourself when to get hungry and when not to get hungry. This is the reason why you can train yourself to get hungry at breakfast or fast for 16 hours plus without food and without feeling any hunger pangs.

One of the reasons fasting works at burning body fat so quickly is due to the hormonal environment it creates. Our bodies are ruled by our hormones. Hormones such as insulin, leptin, testosterone, estrogen, cortisol, ghrelin, thyroid hormone, growth hormone, adrenaline and norepinephrine all play major roles in our moods, how much fat we carry, muscle levels, hunger, satiety, metabolic speed, and more.

Our storage hormone is insulin, and, if we control our insulin levels, we can control whether our body is in fat-storing mode or in fat-burning mode. Whenever we consume carbohydrates, our blood sugar rises and insulin is released to drive blood sugar back to safe levels. Insulin inhibits lipolysis, which is the release of stored triglycerides (body fat).
When we fast, our blood sugar remains stable, which means insulin is not released. This in turn means we're able to access our own fat stores for energy use.

In addition, we make the most use of high cortisol levels in the morning, which further helps break down and mobilise fat. Cortisol can be quite beneficial to fat loss but ONLY in the absence of insulin.

The catecholamines, adrenaline, and norepinephrine are also released in the later hours of the fast. This massively helps increase your metabolic rate as well as access and burn stubborn body fat from around your hips, belly and thigh areas. In the absence of food, growth hormone levels skyrocket, further helping to break down fat tissue and conserve muscle mass.

During fasting, our hormonal environment is optimised to do one thing, and that is to burn body fat fast!

Chapter 3: Dispelling Food and Diet Myths

Let's dispel some of the popular myths surrounding weight loss while answering many of the questions you may have.

Myth #1: Breakfast is the Most Important Meal of the Day

One of the most prevalent myths is that breakfast is the most important meal of the day. I'm sure this is what food companies would like us to believe as there is a whole industry that has been built around breakfast food. Well the short answer is no. Eating breakfast is not critical to your day.

Eating breakfast has no direct impact on weight loss at all. A recent study published in the American Journal of Clinical Nutrition has proven that: whether you have a massive breakfast or if you skip it all together, it doesn't matter. What matters is overall calorie intake for the day.

If you are not hungry when you wake up, it makes sense to simply skip breakfast. Our bodies will efficiently and effectively regulate blood sugar levels and energy levels in the absence of food through a series of metabolic and hormonal processes. When it comes to fat loss, skipping breakfast is not only "not bad" for you, but it is actually a great habit to develop for relatively effortless weight loss.

Myth #2: Don't Eat Before Bed

Another outdated food myth repeated often is to not eat before bed because supposedly the unused energy will go into fat storage. This is also false. There is absolutely no evidence which supports the theory that calories consumed at one time of the day will have more of a tendency to be stored as body fat over calories from a different time of day. Again, I want to reiterate that what does matter is your overall calorie intake for the day.

An appropriate analogy would be the time of day that you top off the fuel in your car. The time of day that the car is refuelled has absolutely no impact on how far you can travel on that tank.

Myth #3: Eating Every 2-3 Hours Increases Your Metabolic Rate

But what about your metabolism? I hear this question all the time when discussing fasting. Aren't you supposed to eat every 2-3 hours to increase metabolic rate? Doesn't skipping meals damage your metabolism? Short answer: no. Long answer: This is quite possibly the most frequently repeated piece of nutritional misinformation out there.

This myth is derived from the thermic effect of food, which is basically the calories burned in order to process the food you eat. The thermic effect of food is approximately 10% of a typical diet. So every time you eat, your metabolic rate increases slightly due to the thermic effect of food (TEF). This process grew into a theory that eating small meals more often would inflate the number of metabolic spikes from TEF, thereby increasing our metabolism and burning more fat. Sounds valid right? Wrong!

Let's take a closer look. Assume we have 2 test subjects, Subject A and Subject B, who each consume the same 3000 calories. Subject A has their 3000 calories divided up into 6 small meals of 500 calories each and Subject B consumes their 3000 calories in 3 large meals of 1000 calories each.

After 6 small meals at 500 calories each, Subject A has a TEF of 50 calories per meal. Multiply this by 6 meals, and we get a total TEF of 300 calories per day.

After 3 large meals of 1000 calories per meal, Subject B has a TEF of 100 calories per meal. Multiply this by 3 meals, and Person B also has a total TEF of 300 calories per day.

The TEF for both Subject A and Subject B are exactly the same.

Myth #4: Skipping Meals Makes Your Metabolism Slow Down

Myth 3 leads us right into myth 4 - a food myth that claims "skipping meals will cause your metabolism to slow down." Yet another false statement. Most studies agree that metabolic down-regulation does not start until approximately 72 hours without food.

Interestingly, at some points during a fast, metabolism can actually speed up due to the release of adrenaline and norepinephrine. This normally occurs at the 20 hours plus mark. The defining line between a fast and starvation is when the fast lasts longer than 72 hours or 3 days. It's important to remember this distinction. Starvation is certainly not healthy, and is not recommended on this plan.

Myth #5: If You Don't Exercise, You Won't Lose Weight

Fitness is a huge trend nowadays. There are social media sites, articles, and an entire fitness culture dedicated to making you believe that exercise is absolutely necessary for weight loss and that not working out will, in turn, cause you to gain weight.

To be clear, lack of exercise does NOT make someone eat the excess food that causes weight gain.

The only way we put on fat is through excess food (calories) intake, NOT the absence of exercise. In general, people today deliberately exercise far more than they did 70 years ago, but are dangerously much more overweight than their predecessors.

Coming from a personal training background, it may seem odd for me not to include an exercise component in this plan and I do love training, don't get me wrong. Exercise however is a large and sticky subject with many variables. Put simply, exercise is unnecessary when dieting effectively. Exercise can also tend to be more of a hindrance in the way that it will make you hungrier. Move more and it's only natural that you will want to eat more.

Exercise is great for building muscle (improving body shape) as well as general physical and mental health. Strategic exercise can assist with weight loss, but should not be viewed as essential to weight loss.

Chapter 4: Fasting Benefits for Your Body and Mind

I've mentioned before that weight loss is more of a mental challenge than a physical one. It's tough trying to figure out which diet and exercise plan will work this time when so many others may have failed you in the past. There could be any number of reasons why those regimens may not have worked for you, but the main one is discipline.

One of the reasons fasting is so effective in producing incredibly fast weight loss results is the self-discipline that you gain and cultivate. Self-control and discipline are like muscles which grow stronger with use. The more you fast, the stronger your self-discipline muscle becomes. As your self-discipline strengthens, sticking to your weight loss plan and focusing on your goals becomes much easier.

The self-discipline achieved from fasting does tend to crossover and benefit other areas of your life as well, such as work, family, relationships, and finances. Many people comment that after starting fasting they feel more empowered and confident that they can take on more of life's challenges. This increase in self-discipline is another reason why fasting becomes almost effortless over time and is a perfect long-term solution for your weight control.

Fasting also tends to shine a spotlight on your eating habits. It teaches you to differentiate between true physical hunger and everything else - cravings, eating out of boredom, and emotional eating such as eating when upset, sad or angry. This can be extremely powerful and eye-opening as well as transformative for people with unhealthy eating habits.

Another major benefit of fasting is that it simplifies and minimises the number of decisions we have to make around food. Everyone has experienced decision fatigue. Have you ever noticed that after making a lot of tough decisions that your ability to continue to make good decisions is lessened?

Consider this, would you be more likely to give in to a burger and fries on a Friday night after a tough work week filled with many tough decisions or on a Sunday evening after a relaxing weekend? Most people would agree they'd be more likely to make the bad decision on a Friday evening after their "decision-making bank account" had been drained.

Having to only make decisions about what to eat healthfully once or twice a day has the amazing benefit of clearing up a massive amount of decision-making bandwidth. The simplicity of this eating plan is freeing. You're not looking at the clock every 2-3 hours like other diet plans and conditioning yourself to constantly think about food. Simply knowing that you're not going to eat until a certain time leaves your mind free to concentrate on other more important tasks.

At the start of fasting, it's quite common to experience a slow, foggy, easily irritable mental state. I'm sure everyone has experienced that grumpy hungry feeling. It's important to bear in mind that this is temporary, and as your body adapts, the true benefits will come to light soon enough.
My clients usually report that, after weeks 1 and 2, they experience vast improvements in their mood, mental clarity, and a sense of well-being. Others have even claimed to feel euphoric. The reason for this may be related to an evolutionary adaptive mechanism during periods without food. Our bodies release chemicals such as adrenaline, norepinephrine, and dopamine when without food. These chemicals give us a happy and calm but alert feeling.

Fasting has a tendency to magnify our emotions. You may initially consider this to be a negative effect, but it can be quite positive as it provides a very real and instant opportunity for internal growth.

Emotions which surface during fasting are often forceful and intense. In such cases I recommend turning attention inward to analyse and correct the thoughts which led to the emotion before they are acted upon.

Most people notice that they feel calmer, clearer, happier and more focused on achieving their goals while practising fasting. The insights and self-improvement gained from this process are factors in why fasting plays such a large role in most major religions.

Fasting is a complete lifestyle change. The specific fasting regimen that follows is more a pattern of eating than a diet. This is often why people find it much easier to make it a permanent part of their lives than typical diets. This is important because losing the weight is easy. Keeping it off is real the challenge.

Fasting is very different to many traditional diets. Most diets sound easy in theory but tend to be hard to practise. Fasting sounds difficult in theory but is actually quite easy to practise. Once you've adapted to fasting, it tends to take on a life of its own. It will begin to feel like the most natural and normal style of eating as long as you don't fight it.

Chapter 5: The Strategy

The nuts and bolts of this plan are simple. There is no calorie counting or macronutrient tracking. You just need to eat intuitively during your eating window and obey your bodily signals of fullness.

Be prepared, invest in a good quality stainless steel water bottle, and always keep it with you. Remember, planning combined with determination is the key to your success!

Step 1. Photos

The first thing you need to do is take your "before" photos. Either take your own selfies or have someone do it for you. Dress in close-fitting, light-coloured clothes, and take full body shots from the front, side, and back. These photos will become priceless to you over the next 1 – 2 months so make sure they are clear, good quality, and show your full body. DO NOT SKIP THIS STEP!

Step 2. Measurements

Take your waist measurement while breathing normally. Make sure that the measuring tape is horizontal and aligned with your belly button.

Step 3. Meal Planning

Plan your meals ahead of time and buy at least 90% of your foods from the lists below. Know what you're going to eat and when you're going to eat, it's crucial. Our sensible decision-making part of the brain tends to get duller, the hungrier we get, so always have a healthy meal available when you are ready to break your fast.

Step 4. Have a Back-Up Plan

You need to have a back-up plan for the tough times. There are going to be difficult periods of time when adapting to any new eating plan, and fasting is no different. Always having back-up food on hand such as almonds or anything else in the allowed list is important.

Step 5. Don't Overtrain

Limit training to 2 -3 days a week at most while following this eating plan. Let this eating plan do the heavy lifting when it comes to fat loss. When training, focus more on resistance training than on intense cardio.

Chapter 6: The Fast

Your fast will start from the time of your last meal before you go to sleep up until your first meal 16 hours later (at least). Upon waking drink at least 500 ml of water. This will help ward off any possible breakfast hunger.

The Eating Window
Once your 16 hours are up, do an assessment of your "physical hunger levels" using the following hunger level scale.

7 – Stuffed: You are so full you feel sick and physical pain.

6 - Very uncomfortably full: You need to loosen your clothes.

5 - Uncomfortably full: You feel bloated and have that "heavy" feeling.

4 – Full: You feel a little bit uncomfortable, starting to feel "heavy".

3 - Comfortable: You're satisfied. Not hungry, still feel light, unconcerned about food.

2 – Slightly hungry: You're just beginning to physically feel signs of hunger. Thoughts about food are likely to arise. This is your first sign to start drinking lots of water.

1 – Real hunger: Your stomach is churning/tummy is rumbling.

If after 16 hours of fasting you find yourself at:

Level 1 hunger - then it's fine to eat at 16 hours.
Level 2 hunger - then try and push your meal out for another 1-2 hours.
Level 3 hunger - then try and delay your meal for another 2-3 hours.

Once you decide to break your fast you will enter your "eating window". In your eating window, eat one large meal and one small meal. Your 2 meals should be as far apart as possible and there should be no snacking between meals.

To maintain somewhat of a routine (and because there are only 24 hours in a day), keep in mind that as your fasts get longer, your eating window will get shorter.

For fasts over 20 hours, it is fine to eat just one large meal during your eating window. Just make sure not to overeat (i.e. Level 5 on the hunger scale and above).

When starting out with 16 hour fasts your eating window would be a time period of 8 hours. Within those 8 hours you would consume 2 meals. Meal timings could be at hours 16 and hour 24 or of your own choosing.

On a longer fast like 20 hours then you would have an eating window of 4 hours that you could either eat 2 meals (possibly at hours 20 and 24) or 1 large meal (at hour 20).

Getting started

The easiest way to approach a 16-hour fast when starting out is by simply skipping breakfast and having a late lunch. Here's how your day may look like on a typical 16-hour fast.

Last meal the previous night eaten at 8pm.

Meal 1 would be eaten at 12pm. A fibrous, low-calorie meal is important if you find yourself ravenous after the fast , preferably containing green vegetables. This could include a salad, steamed vegetables, boiled eggs, or a can of tuna.

Meal 2 would be eaten between 6pm and 8pm. This would be a smaller-sized meal than meal 1 and would likely be meat and vegetable based, e.g. sausages with roast vegetables.

Phase 1

For the first 3 weeks, while your body is adapting, aim for a minimum 16-hour fast every day. If you notice that by the 16-hour mark, you are consistently not hungry, try to push your fast to 20 hours plus. The 20-hour plus mark is generally the sweet spot for most people. Here they will see the most dramatic weight loss results in the shortest time.

Phase 2

After 4 weeks of daily fasting, reduce your fasts to 5 days per week. You will take 2 days off a week, and switch back to a 3-meal-a-day eating pattern with the same foods during your off days. At first, you may notice that you're not hungry at the normal breakfast and lunch times, but making yourself eat a small meal at these times helps reset hormonal processes in the body. It also ensures that you will continue to get results throughout the week.

You will find that after 2 consecutive days of eating 3 meals a day you may feel extremely hungry again at those same times in the following days. This is EXACTLY what we want. We want to continually be one step ahead of our body adapting to our weight loss routine. The fact that you feel hungry again during the day while fasting is a sure sign of continued weight loss.

Continue this regimen of fasting for 16-20 hours for 5 days and eating at normal times for 2 days out of the week. If necessary, you can spread the "normal meal days" apart. You know your body best and can determine which method is the most effective for you.

Weigh yourself on the same day once a week during both phases. Make sure that you always weigh yourself under the same conditions, i.e. First thing in the morning in same clothes after a toilet stop.

Do NOT be affected by the number on the scale. There are many factors to consider when it comes to scale weight so pay more attention to what's happening in the mirror and how your clothes fit.

Maintenance

The same eating plan that got you the results will need to be the same to the eating plan you use to maintain those results (or very similar).

Eating for maintenance is going to look slightly different for different people depending on their body type and eating history. The best advice I can offer is below in combination with following your own body's feedback.

General Maintenance Guidelines:

If you have an endomorph body type, have a history of weight problems, and have a lot of weight to lose then you will more than likely need to stay on a strict carb-controlled style of eating combined with longer daily fasts 5-6 days a week to maintain goal weight.

If you have more of an ectomorph body type, and have been mostly lean in your past…
Then continue fasting, but decrease to 3 – 4 days of fasting per week and keep carbohydrates under 160 gms per day.

For those with a mesomorph body type, and no major history of weight problems…Continue with daily fasting 4-5 days a week and keep carbohydrates intake to under 120 gms per day.

In general, your meals should be protein dominant with moderate fat levels and lower in carbohydrates. Acceptable cuisines could include Indian, Thai, Japanese, and Malaysian curries, roast meats, roasted vegetables, salads, casseroles, soups, barbecued and grilled meats, cold meat, and salads. Below is a list of acceptable foods, foods to be enjoyed in moderation, and foods to avoid while following this eating plan.

Allowed Foods (everyday foods)

Bacon
Beef (Preferably grass-fed)
Chicken
Crab
Duck
Lamb
Mackerel
Pork
Prawns
Salmon
Sardines
Traditionally-Prepared Meat (Chorizo and Kielbasa)
Tuna
Turkey
Veal
Eggs: (Free-range is preferable)
Vegetables: All above-ground, non-starchy, non-root vegetables are allowed. Frozen forms of the listed vegetables are also acceptable.
Asian Greens
Broccoli
Brussel Sprouts
Cabbage
Capsicum
Cauliflower

Cucumber
Eggplant
Garlic
Lettuce
Onion
Spinach
Zucchini
Pumpkin
Spices and Herbs: Enjoy as much as you want as long as they are free from additives and artificial flavourings.
Healthy Fats and Oils
Butter
Coconut Milk & Cream
Coconut Oil
Ghee
Olive Oil
Condiments
 Fish Sauce
Mayonnaise
Mustards
Oyster Sauce
Pesto
Salsa
Soy Sauce
Tomato Sauces and Pastes, Low-Sugar
Vinegars (Apple Cider and Balsamic)
Avocadoes
Blueberries
Strawberries

Allowed, In Moderation (2-3 nights per week)

Starchy Vegetables and Root Vegetables
Limit the intake of these foods to a maximum of 3 nights per week. For better results, save them for one night on the weekend.
Beetroots
Carrots
Cassava
Potatoes
Sweet Potatoes
Taro
Dairy: Although most people do not have reactions to dairy, it can be slightly insulinogenic despite relatively low carbs, and, therefore, should be limited. For best results, limit intake to 1 night a week max.
Butter
Cheeses
Creams
Milk
Yogurts
Natural Sweeteners: Honey, Maple Syrup (limit to 2 times a week max.)
Nuts and Seeds: These are extremely calorie dense and are often "trigger" foods for many people. They also contain mostly omega-6 fats of which most people already have too much of in their diets. Limit consumption to 2 nights a week max.
Cashews
Macadamia
Peanuts
Rice (White or Brown): High in carbs and calories so do limit consumption to 2-3 times per week max.

Fruits: Try to minimise these if super-fast fat loss is desired. Limit to 2 nights per week.

Apples
Bananas
Coconuts
Grapes
Mangoes
Melons
Pears
Watermelon

Dried Fruits: Be very careful with these as they are not as filling as regular fruit but have just as many calories. Beware of additives such as seed oils. Limit to 1 night per week.

Apricots
Dates
Prunes
Sultanas

Alcohol: Stick to spirits without sugary mixers, e.g. Vodka lime and sodas, gin and tonic, whiskey on the rocks. When drinking wine, choose a non-sweet, non-sparkling version like a dry red. Limit consumption to 1 – 2 nights per week of a maximum of 4 standard drinks.

Do NOT Eat

Grains and Whole Grains: There are many reasons to avoid these foods, however, the most important are: anti-nutrients and carbohydrate content.
Breads
Pita Bread
Corn
Couscous
Oats
Pasta
Rye
Semolina
Wheat
Legumes: Although not as bad as grains, they are on the banned list for the same reasons – anti-nutrients such as Phytates and Lectins. The one exception to this rule would be if you are a vegetarian.
Beans, Broad
Beans, Canellini
Beans, Fava
Beans, Kidney
Beans, Lima
Chickpeas
Lentils
Soybeans
Refined Sugars and Artificial Sweeteners - Anything containing both real sugars and artificial sweeteners, such as chocolates, bakery products, ice cream, soft drinks.
Pre-packaged and Processed Foods - Canned is generally acceptable if it contains only one ingredient.
Seed Oils and Unhealthy Fats
Margarine
Oil, Canola
Oil, Soybean
Oil, Vegetable
Junk Food - This includes but is not limited to French fries, pies, pizza, sausage rolls, and packaged foods.

Chapter 8: Hunger Busters!

You should expect your hunger levels to fluctuate up and down throughout the day during your fast. You need to be prepared for this and have a plan in place for when hunger pangs strike hard. Use these "Hunger Busters" in the following order to defeat cravings, and untimely hunger.

1. Water
This is your most powerful hunger-busting tool. In fact it's so powerful that your success or failure is nearly dependent on this. Training yourself to drink water the instant a thought or feeling of hunger arises is of utmost importance. Use water at any time of the day. It will help keep you full, ward off hunger and keep your weight loss constant.

Aim for 2-3 litres of water per day or until your urine runs clear. Invest in a good quality stainless steel water bottle, and always keep it close by.
This first step alone is often enough to ward off 70-90% of your hunger signals during this eating plan.

2. Black Coffee and Green Tea
This is the second most powerful tool to combat hunger. Black coffee and green tea should only be used if your hunger levels are unable to be controlled by water alone. Black coffee and green tea, without any sweeteners, artificial sweeteners, or milk, should be used sparingly and strategically during a fast.

Green tea is preferable due to it's longer-lasting energy curve and increased benefits from higher levels of antioxidants. Moreover, green tea also has a strong effect on the catecholamines, which signals your fat cells to release fat into the bloodstream for use as energy.

Tea and black coffee help blunt hunger and are great energy boosters since you may experience low energy as a normal part of adjusting to this fasting plan. However, keep in mind that, if used excessively (5+ cups or tea or coffee per day), the increased fat burning and appetite suppressant effects of the fast can be lost. Limit yourself to a maximum of 3 strong cups of black coffee and/or green tea per day, and do not drink them after 2pm as the caffeine can affect your sleep quality and fat loss results.

Not everyone enjoys the flavour of black coffee so, if you fall in this category, I have a couple of tips to help make it more palatable.

Change the way you think of coffee. View it more as a tool to get you to your goal and not something that should taste good. Also try:

- Try consuming coffee shots – smaller quantity, stronger dose
- Try consuming cold coffee as opposed to hot coffee

3. Steamed Green Vegetables and Miso Soup
This is your very last resort. It should only be used if absolutely necessary during the first 1-2 weeks. They both contain some calories so are best avoided since a true fast, for our purposes, needs to have 0 calories. However, if it's between this option and ruining your weight loss plan by binge eating, then eating some steamed vegetables or a miso soup is the preferred option.

Chapter 9: Do's and Don'ts
"Do's"

DO Drink LOTS of Water. This is the a key factor to your success. Drink lots of water. You should be taking in a minimum of 2 litres per day, and 3 litres is even better. Your urine should run clear. There will be many toilet stops at first, but, as your body adjusts to the increased water intake, the urge to visit the toilet will lessen. Drinking lots of water has been repeated many times throughout this book for good reason. If you feel you aren't going to make it to 16 hours, the first thing you should do is skoll 2 large glasses of water. Usually, the water and a little distraction is all you need to fend off the most intense hunger pains.

DO Use the Deadline Dieting "Hunger Buster" strategies (Outlined Above)

DO Stay Busy. Time moves slower the more you pay attention to it, so if you find yourself constantly checking the clock, do yourself a favour and distract yourself by doing something productive. Time will fly by and it will be dinner time in no time!

DO Practise food mindfulness. Stop thinking about food all the time! Easier said than done I know, especially when hungry. This is an important point however. Try not to allow yourself to be consumed by the thought of food or how much time is left until your next meal. Our thoughts often lead to actions, therefore its best not to even entertain food thoughts. This ties in to the previous point of staying busy and finding something to override any thoughts of food. Thoughts, like stress, have a very specific effect on the human body. Studies have shown that fantasising about food stimulates insulin secretion in anticipation of food. Our goal is to create a hormonal environment that

DO Keep a "Motivation & Inspiration Folder" a collection of images of your goal body type. This could be a folder of images on your phone or computer of celebrities, models, fitness models, or photos of yourself when you were at your goal weight. Use these images to motivate and keep you on track during the tough times. To keep these images "front of mind" set yourself a reminder for every Sunday to go over them to keep motivation levels high. This time should also be used to add motivational images and personal notes to the folder as well.

DO Keep trying. When starting this eating plan, achieving 16 hour daily fasts consistently is your number one goal. There may be times when you don't reach 16hours. Don't be discouraged or look at it as a failure. Simply learn from your experience and try again tomorrow. There are always going to be tough days where your hunger hits a level 1 at only 10 or 11 hours into a fast when new to fasting. These are the challenging times you will need to push through in order to get results. Self-analyse and pay attention to the thought processes that cut any fasts short. Was the reason mental or physical? Has this same thought patterns caused you to give in before? Did you follow the hunger buster steps? Correct course and strive to do better the next day.

"Don'ts"

DON'T Consume Calories During Your Fast. Do not take in any liquid calories, other than when absolutely necessary and as defined by our "Hunger Busters" section, and, of course, do not take in solid calories at all.

DON'T Inhale Your First Meal of the Day. Take your time. Savour your food. Many of you will be extremely hungry following your fast, but this is all about self-discipline and self-control. If you gorge on your first meal, you risk overeating and consuming an overabundance of calories. Overeating at just one meal has the potential to undo all of the progress from one day of fasting, and, if it's a full on binge, it could reverse an entire week of work. To overcome this, break your fast with a small light meal, such as a salad, some steamed vegetables, or a protein shake. Make sure to eat slowly, since it takes about 20 minutes for your brain to register a feeling of fullness, and stop eating once you are about 80% full.

DON'T Be afraid of higher fat intake. If your carbohydrate intake is low then it is quite healthy and recommended to eat higher levels of fat. Yes even saturated fat (most often seen in animal meat and products). The latest evidence in scientific research has found no link between saturated fat and heart disease. For more information on this topic I recommend the hugely popular book - Good Calories, Bad Calories by Gary Taubes.

DON'T Give up. Learn from any past bad days and don't repeat the same mistakes. The will to continue and improve day by day is what matters most. Strive for consistency.

DON'T Eat anything outside of the "allowed" and "in Moderation" food groups   This is important even if the food is considered to be "healthy". Our primary goal is fat loss and improved health is an automatic side effect. There are many so called health foods that are simply too high in calories or carbs to be of any use during a weight loss program. Foods on the "allowed" and "in moderation" lists simply work for fat loss. Results cannot be guaranteed if other foods are introduced.

Chapter 10: Plateaus

Let's talk about plateaus. They are real, frustrating and a likely part of your weight loss journey. Some plateaus can last 1 -2 weeks. Others can last as long as 1 – 2 months. What's important is that you do NOT let it affect your mindset.
Be prepared for it. Everyone can push through plateaus. It's a good idea to return to basics if you find yourself within a plateau. Make sure you are doing everything perfectly including foods from allowed list, not eating past satisfaction, and taking 2 days off from fasting per week.

At the end of the plateau you will almost certainly experience the "whoosh effect,". The "whoosh" effect is a sudden drop of 1-2 kg (2-4 lbs). The most plausible theory explaining this phenomenon is that as fat cells empty of stored triglycerides they temporarily refill with water. This is likely due to the fact that glycerol which is the backbone of fatty acids attracts water. After the water is finally released, the fat cells shrink and weight loss becomes noticeable.

Chapter 11: Food Mindfulness - Vigilance is Victory

You are not your thoughts and your food thoughts only have as much weight as you give them.

Bear in mind that at any one point in time there could be 10 different thoughts playing on repeat in the back of our minds. These thoughts are e not us until we attach ourselves to them and act upon them.

These thoughts often don't even align with our beliefs or goals but will still make up the background noise in our heads.

Thoughts grow in strength the more they are thought and these thoughts lead to action.The best way to interrupt these non-serving thought patterns is to crowd them out with good, results-inspiring thoughts and images.

Practise catching yourself anytime you find that you are playing out old, negative, food-related thought patterns. Replace these thoughts with visions of you already having achieved you goal body. To act on food cravings would then be to risk losing something you already have. This can be an effective technique to always stay on track. The motivating pain of loss is usually stronger than the desire of attainment.

Practising "food mindfulness" is of extreme importance to the success or failure of your fasting.

Pay close attention to what thoughts are playing in the back of your mind while fasting. If they are food-related, get rid of them entirely during your fast. Once the dieting mind is controlled I promise you that fat loss results through fasting will become ever more effortless.

Chapter 12: One Last Thing

There are some other exciting benefits to fasting that I've been saving until the end to tell you about. Would you be interested in looking younger, living longer, and being healthier overall with improved mood and brain function? Well who wouldn't be right?

Well it's long been known that long-term caloric restriction of around 30 -40% below maintenance has some major benefits to our health. These benefits include improved blood sugar regulation, lower insulin concentration and insulin-related substances such as insulin-like growth factor 1 and lower blood pressure.

These factors directly lead to living longer and looking younger. However, ask anyone who's been on a low-calorie diet, however, and they will tell you that it's not exactly a pleasant experience. The downsides are mood swings, irritability, hostility and depression.

The good news is that the very latest scientific research studies have found that the same health benefits of caloric restriction can be achieved through a different method – Fasting! You experience the same benefits but with more calories and less downsides.

What the animal studies did was compare a group of animals who were put on a fasting regime and a second group who ate half the amount of calories but at whatever time they wanted. What the researchers found was that the group of animals who were on the fasting regime displayed all of the same health benefits observed on calorie-restricted diet but ate twice as many calories at their designated meal time!

The reason for this, researchers explained, is due to a process called autophagy. Autophagy is a cellular process that happens in all living cells during low-energy states, such as fasting and caloric restriction. Autophagy literally means "self-consumption". It is basically when our cells "eat themselves", clean house and recycle the trash. It allows the defective, damaged and unwanted parts of our cells which cause aging and disease to be cleared out.

Autophagy also explains why we see beneficial effects from green tea, resveratrol (from red wine), exercise, caffeine, as they all trigger this process to a certain degree.

A defective and inadequate autophagy response is now agreed to be the major driver behind aging and aging related diseases. There is much more evidence in support of autophagy activation as a viable way to promote longevity and slow aging than in any other protocol, such as hormone replacement, supplementation, or telomerase or stem cell therapy. Plus, autophagy activation through fasting is free and readily available to anyone at any time.

Another exciting find in the fasted animal group was an increase in brain-derived neurotrophic factor (BDNF) levels. BDNF promotes new neuron growth, repairs failing brain cells, and protects healthy brain cells. Increased BDNF in humans translates to easier acquisition and retention of new knowledge, and a happier state of mind. In fact, increased BDNF is thought to be one of the primary reasons antidepressants, such as Prozac, work so effectively. BDNF also improves insulin sensitivity, which is great for fat loss.

So, there you have it! "Eating yourself" for breakfast and lunch is now known to be one of the best things you can do not only to lose weight and stay lean but also to live a long healthy, happy, and productive life.

Chapter 13: Say Hello to the New You!

"Happiness is not something ready-made, it comes from your own actions"- Dalai Lama

Mental strength is an often neglected aspect of most diets and usually not even mentioned. This is an area where fasting stands apart from other eating plans. Fasting provides a real opportunity for internal and external improvement quickly. The personal growth combined with an effective eating plan can be life- transforming.

From my experience in training and coaching clients over the years, I've come to realise that a client's short-term success depends on their mindset and their willingness to work hard while following a given program 100%. Being able to push through the tough times of a diet is truly the difference between getting "so-so" results and achieving a body others are going to be jealous of.

Long-term sustainable weight loss is due to changing one's thoughts and habits around food while following a specific framework.

I therefore encourage you to adopt fasting as a part of your new lifestyle. Remember, weight loss is a marathon, not a sprint. Weight loss should be transformational internally and externally. It can be one of your greatest joys and achievements or it could be a tortuous 12 weeks of pain and discomfort.

You now have the knowledge and power to choose which one it will be through your mindset and attitude towards this eating plan.

If you fully embrace this eating plan as part of a healthy and slim lifestyle, you will continually see remarkable health benefits and look amazing with minimal effort.

I've seen the results with both myself and many clients. I am certain the "Deadline Dieting" plan can be the most successful weight loss plan you've tried yet and the last plan you'll ever need. So say goodbye to diets and say hello to the new you!

www.ingramcontent.com/pod-product-compliance
Lightning Source LLC
Chambersburg PA
CBHW070232290526
45789CB00004B/1591